Ivianne Ortiz Sotolongo
Marcilia Cabrera Copa
Perla M Trujillo Pedroza

Educational program on cerebrovascular diseases

Ivianne Ortiz Sotolongo
Marcilia Cabrera Copa
Perla M Trujillo Pedroza

Educational program on cerebrovascular diseases

Impact on patients at risk

ScienciaScripts

Imprint
Any brand names and product names mentioned in this book are subject to trademark, brand or patent protection and are trademarks or registered trademarks of their respective holders. The use of brand names, product names, common names, trade names, product descriptions etc. even without a particular marking in this work is in no way to be construed to mean that such names may be regarded as unrestricted in respect of trademark and brand protection legislation and could thus be used by anyone.

Cover image: www.ingimage.com

This book is a translation from the original published under ISBN 978-613-9-46600-9.

Publisher:
Sciencia Scripts
is a trademark of
Dodo Books Indian Ocean Ltd. and OmniScriptum S.R.L publishing group

120 High Road, East Finchley, London, N2 9ED, United Kingdom
Str. Armeneasca 28/1, office 1, Chisinau MD-2012, Republic of Moldova, Europe
Printed at: see last page
ISBN: 978-620-8-30973-2

TITLE:

EDUCATIONAL PROGRAMME ON CEREBROVASCULAR DISEASES.

IMPACT ON PATIENTS AT RISK

AUTHORS:

DR. IVIANNE ORTIZ SOTOLONGO.

THIRD YEAR RESIDENT IN THE SPECIALITY OF GENERAL COMPREHENSIVE MEDICINE.

DR. MARCILIA CABRERA COPA.

1ST DEGREE SPECIALIST IN INTERNAL MEDICINE. ASSISTANT PROFESSOR. MASTER IN INFECTIOUS DISEASES.

DR. PERLA M. TRUJILLO PEDROZA

1ST DEGREE SPECIALIST IN MGI. MASTER IN PHC. ASSISTANT PROFESSOR. ASSOCIATE RESEARCHER

2024

SUMMARY

Cerebrovascular disease, cerebrovascular accident or stroke, is a complex age-related disease with high mortality and long-term disability. In Cuba, it is the third leading cause of death. From January to December 2023, a quasi-experimental intervention study was conducted to assess the impact of an educational programme in patients with risk factors for cerebrovascular disease. Of the population between 50 and 60 years of age dispensed in the clinic

11 as risk of cerebrovascular disease a sample of 35 patients was selected by non-probability sampling by criteria. A predominance of the male sex was observed for 54.3 % and the age group 55-60 years. The main risk factor found was hypertension with 30 patients, followed by diabetes mellitus, 85.7 % and 51.4 % respectively. In the study, 27 patients had inadequate knowledge of the types of stroke and after the Educational Programme was applied, the figures decreased, with only 6 patients showing inadequate knowledge. After implementation of the programme 88.6 % had adequate knowledge of the risk factors. At the end of the intervention, 45.7% and 71.4% had better control of diabetes mellitus and hypertension, respectively. The application of the Educational Programme: "Stroke in the 21st century" had a favourable impact on the study sample.

TABLE OF CONTENTS

INTRODUCTION

Cerebrovascular disease, cerebrovascular accident or stroke, is a complex age-related disease with high mortality and long-term disability. (1) Cerebrovascular diseases are a group of conditions of the cerebral vasculature resulting from an occlusion or rupture of an extra vessel in the brain. This leads to a decrease in cerebral blood flow with consequent transient or permanent impairment of the function of a generalised region of the brain or a smaller or focal area. [(2)]

The history of cerebrovascular disease is very ancient. [(3)] In antiquity, beginning with remote cultures such as Sumerian-Babylonian, Egyptian and Hebrew, there are suggestive descriptions of stroke. Thus, in the Bible, they are written in the Book of Psalms, where King David exclaims: "Let my right hand be forgotten, and let my tongue cleave to the roof of my mouth". Likewise, in the historical era of medicine, quotations concerning stroke appear in papyri written by Edwin Smith around 1550 BC, in Herodotus' book of history, in writings left by Diogenes, as well as in Hippocrates' Treatise on Medicine in about 460-370 BC.[(4)] Hippocrates, considered the Father of Medicine, recognised and wrote, to the pride of Neurologists, about stroke more than 2,400 years ago.[(3)] In 1620, the Swiss Johann Wepfer was the first to identify brain signs in patients who died of stroke, indicating that stroke, in addition to being caused by haemorrhage in the brain, could also be caused by blockage of one of the main arteries supplying blood to the brain. In time, Wepfer's hypothesis would be confirmed. [(5)]

The World Health Organisation classifies stroke as ischaemic or haemorrhagic. The former is caused by an obstruction of a blood vessel, and the latter by rupture, resulting in intracerebral haemorrhage. [(6)] Sixty percent of strokes of these events occur outside the hospital. Approximately 87% of cerebrovascular events are ischaemic and 13% haemorrhagic, and although the former is the most frequent, the latter has the highest mortality, with in-hospital mortality described as 5-10% and 40-60% respectively. [(7)]

The risk of cerebrovascular disease depends largely on the occurrence of risk factors, which are classified as non-modifiable and modifiable. The Framingham study highlights risk factors such as dyslipidaemia; high blood pressure which doubles the risk; smoking; diabetes mellitus which increases the likelihood of developing cardiovascular disease by two to three times; physical inactivity; hyperglycaemia with values above 180 mg/dl or 10 mmol/l; oral contraceptives increase platelet aggregation increasing the possibility of clot formation. [(8)]

High blood pressure is the most important risk factor for both cerebral ischaemia and cerebral haemorrhage, being found in almost 70% of stroke patients. The risk of stroke increases proportionally with blood pressure in both men and women, and in all age groups. 15-20% of ischaemic strokes are cardioembolic in origin, with atrial fibrillation accounting for almost 50% of all cases, a common pathology whose prevalence increases with age.(9)

According to the World Health Organisation, 15 million people worldwide have a stroke each year, 5.5 million of whom die and another 5 million are left with a permanent disability(10,11) , making it the third leading cause of death in industrialised countries (after cardiovascular diseases and cancer). The disease is said to increase in incidence after the age of 60, when atherosclerotic processes reach their peak(12) . It is the most common cause of neurological disability in adults and the most likely in women. people over 65 years of age; this situation affects both high-income and developing countries. (3)

The global incidence of stroke is 200 cases per 100,000 inhabitants/year and a 27% increase in the incidence of stroke is expected between 2000 and 2025, related to the ageing of the population. (13) The age-adjusted incidence of stroke in Europe has been estimated to be between 95 and 290/100,000 inhabitants per year. Approximately 1.1 million Europeans suffer a stroke each year; 80% of these cases are ischaemic strokes. Between 20-35% of patients die within the first month after a stroke, and approximately one third of the survivors lose their autonomy. (14)

Mortality rates of 61.5/100 000 inhabitants are reported in developed countries such as the United States of America, France, Germany and Italy where it is estimated that one stroke event occurs every 53 seconds and one death every 3.3 minutes. (3) In China, an epidemiological survey confirmed that the standardised mortality rate for cerebrovascular disease has reached 120.1 per 100 000 population. (15)

The prevalence of cerebrovascular disease in Latin America is high. (8) In Latin America, the incidence of cerebrovascular disease is reported to be between 0.89-1.83/1000. On the other hand, prevalence figures for cerebrovascular disease range from 1.7 to 6.5 /1000. (16)

In Cuba, cerebrovascular diseases are the third leading cause of death, after cardiovascular diseases and malignant tumours. (3) The Cuban population is ageing, not growing and is likely to decrease. The elderly population is close to 14 %, the incidence of cerebrovascular diseases currently increases with age, and mortality increases exponentially with age, doubling every 5 years. In Cuba, the western and central provinces are the most affected. The risk is higher due to the fact that the population is the oldest in the country. (17) According to the Statistical Yearbook in Cuba in 2019 there were 10 152 deaths with an increase in 2020 of 10 821 deaths for this disease(18) , with a crude rate calculated at 96.6 per 100 000 inhabitants, of which 5 618 deaths were male (crude rate 100.9/10000) and 5203 female (crude rate 92.4/10000), a prevalence of 6.8 per 1000 inhabitants and the average number of years of potential life lost per 1000 inhabitants due to this disease was estimated at 4. (19) At the Hospital Provincial Docente Clinicoquirúrgico Saturnino Lora Torres in Santiago de Cuba, 1 803 patients with a diagnosis of stroke were treated in the period 2016-2021, of which 1 197 (66.3 %) corresponded to ischaemic cerebrovascular disease. (20) In Villa Clara, the prevalence of cerebrovascular diseases in 2020 was 4.8 per 1 000 inhabitants, with 757 deaths, a figure higher than in 2019, when mortality was 668. (18) In the "Marta Abreu" Polyclinic, in 2019, 112 new cases were diagnosed compared to previous years, with an increase in incidence. (3)

In a study carried out by Piloto Cruz at the Central Military Hospital "Dr. Carlos J. Finlay", 54.7 % of the patients were over 70 years of age and 58.7 % were male. Smoking was found in 87.7 % of patients with atherothrombotic stroke. More than 80 % of patients with ischaemic and haemorrhagic strokes were hypertensive. (12)

In the 11th clinic, Manuel Piti Fajardo Polyclinic, Santo Domingo, the annual statistics are similar to those of the rest of the population of Villaclare, where there is a high incidence and prevalence of people with risk factors that increase the development of cerebrovascular diseases in the short or long term. The impact of risk factors for cerebrovascular disease and the scarcity of information on the part of the population has been a crucial motivation for the implementation of an educational programme, and the following scientific problem has arisen: What is the impact of an educational programme on patients with risk factors for cerebrovascular disease at Consultorio No. 11, Santo Domingo, January-December 2023?

Hypothesis: With the application of an educational programme that includes lectures, videos, audiovisuals and participatory techniques in patients with risk factors for cerebrovascular disease, the knowledge of these factors improves and their modification is achieved.

OBJECTIVES

General objective: To assess the impact of an educational programme in patients with risk factors for cerebrovascular disease. Clinic No. 11 Santo Domingo, January - December 2023.

Objectives specific:

1. Distribute the sample according to age and sex.
2. To identify risk factors for cerebrovascular disease according to sex in the population.
3. Design an educational programme on risk factors for cerebrovascular disease.
4. To determine knowledge of cerebrovascular disease, cerebrovascular disease risk factors before and after the intervention in the population.
5. To compare the behaviour of some risk factors before and after the intervention in the study population.

THEORETICAL FRAMEWORK

Cerebrovascular disease. General.

Cerebrovascular disease is a hierarchically broad term. It is a syndrome that includes a group of heterogeneous diseases with one thing in common: a disturbance in the vasculature of the central nervous system, leading to an imbalance between oxygen supply and oxygen requirements.[21] is considered as such all conditions resulting in a transient or permanent brain disorder caused by ischaemia or haemorrhage, secondary to a pathological process of the blood vessels of the brain. [16]

The World Health Organisation defines stroke as "rapidly developing clinical signs of focal (sometimes global) impairment of brain function, lasting more than 24 hours or leading to death with no apparent cause other than vascular origin". An updated definition of central nervous system infarction has been proposed by the American Heart Association / American Stroke Association. Central nervous system infarction (including haemorrhagic infarction) is defined as "damage to the brain, spinal cord, or retinal cell death attributable to ischaemia, based on: pathological, imaging, or other objective evidence of focal cerebral, spinal cord, or retinal ischaemic injury in a defined vascular distribution; or clinical evidence of focal cerebral, spinal cord, or retinal ischaemic injury based on symptoms persisting ≥24 hours or until death, and other aetiologies have been excluded". [22]

Cerebrovascular disease is the leading cause of significant mortality worldwide; it is believed that for every symptomatic stroke there are 9 that occur silently and affect the cognitive level of sufferers; this pathology occurs at any stage of life. [23]

Cases of cerebrovascular disease, in general, have increased in recent years, from the fifth leading cause of disability in 1990 to the third in 2010 alone. [24]

The brain is the organ responsible for processing and storing all information relevant to the functioning of the individual. Without the blood supply, neurons become apoptotic resulting in brain damage. The level of disability varies according to the type of stroke suffered, the part of the brain affected and the size of the damaged area. [25]

Cerebrovascular disease. Classification.

According to the US National Institute of Neurological Disorders and Stroke classification, published in 1990, there are four variants: asymptomatic, vascular dementia, hypertensive encephalopathy and focal cerebral vascular dysfunction. (16)

- Asymptomatic cerebrovascular disease, which has not yet produced brain or retinal symptoms but has caused some demonstrable vascular damage.
- Focal cerebrovascular disease encompassing:

• Transient ischaemic attack: a clinical picture resulting from the focal and transient interruption of the cerebral circulation, without causing necrosis and resulting in neurological deficit for less than 24 hours.

• Cerebral infarction: a neurological condition that occurs when a specific area of the brain dies due to a lack of blood supply, as a result of a clot blocking the lumen of the artery.

• Intracerebral haemorrhage.

• Subarachnoid haemorrhage: is the clinical picture resulting from extravasation of blood into the subarachnoid or leptomeningeal space. It is most often caused by The second common cause is congenital and acquired arterial aneurysms.

- Vascular dementia: any condition that progresses with global deterioration of intellectual functions and is secondary to lesions in the brain parenchyma due to alterations of vascular origin. This condition occurs in 20 of all patients with cerebrovascular diseases and accounts for 15-25% of all dementias.
- Hypertensive encephalopathy: an acute syndrome presenting with severe arterial hypertension, which exceeds the upper limit of autoregulation. It is an acute or subacute consequence of severe hypertension, a potentially reversible brain disorder.

According to their nature, strokes are divided into haemorrhagic and ischaemic[26] , with ischaemic stroke being more frequent at 70% (range: 42-98%), followed by subarachnoid haemorrhage (20%, 0 to 45%), intracerebral haemorrhage (10%, 0 to 29%), and cerebral thrombosis (0.5 to 1%). More than 76% of strokes are primary events; 85% are preventable. [1]

Cerebrovascular disease. Risk factors.

In general terms, the World Health Organisation defines a risk factor as "any trait, characteristic or exposure of an individual that increases his or her likelihood of suffering a disease or injury". Epidemiological studies show that the occurrence of many of the diseases we know does not occur randomly, but that there are many causes involved, which makes it necessary to know the existence and magnitude of the association between these causes and the occurrence of the diseases. [4]

Cerebrovascular disease is a multifactorial disease that manifests itself in the presence of a combination of risk factors, not all of which may be present, but which influence, over time, the likelihood of the person suffering from the condition. [27,28]

The burden of disease that a risk factor generates in the population depends on its prevalence, the strength of the association of the risk factor with the disease and its predictive value. These risk factors are responsible for a very large proportion of cerebrovascular disease in the general population. Moreover, the risk factors are mutually reinforcing and frequently occur in association with each other. [9]

Many risk factors for cerebrovascular disease have been identified: well documented or confirmed modifiable risk factors (hypertension, recent myocardial infarction, smoking, sickle cell anaemia, previous transient ischaemic attacks, asymptomatic carotid stenosis, hypercholesterolemia, alcohol consumption, physical inactivity, obesity, dietary factors, hyperinsulinaemia and insulin resistance), potentially modifiable ones (diabetes mellitus, haemocystinaemia, hypercoagulable states, left ventricular hypertrophy, infections, migraine and subclinical processes), non-modifiable risk factors (age, sex, hereditary factors, ethnicity, geographic location and socio-cultural level), less documented and potentially modifiable risk factors (some heart diseases, oral contraceptive use and drug use) and non-modifiable risk factors (season and climate). [3]

It is important to detect patients with modifiable factors because, although these cannot be treated, it identifies high-risk subjects in whom the coexistence of modifiable factors requires their vigorous control, and they are candidates for other preventive therapies. Therefore, they are distinguished within the most common modifiable factors: [9]

Arterial hypertension: Arterial hypertension is a condition in which blood pressure is constantly elevated with values equal to or above 140 millimetres of mercury (mmHg) of systolic pressure and 90 mmHg of diastolic pressure. It is also considered to be a preventable disease, which is classified as a risk factor for cardiovascular diseases, which are the leading causes of mortality worldwide. This condition damages the perforating arteries responsible for cerebral circulation, which are detached at a ninety-degree angle from the arteries of the cerebral arterial circle. [29] Arterial hypertension, which produces high mortality rates in countries with epidemiological transition, proves to be a major and common diagnosis within coronary heart disease, as well as having an impact on stroke, which is another common cause of death and others that impact on people's quality of life. [30]

It is the major risk factor triggering cerebrovascular disease and worldwide,[29] is present in the majority of patients with ischaemic cerebrovascular disease and in subjects with intracranial haemorrhage[31] , in which the malignant form of arterial hypertension is the frequent antecedent (78% to 88%) .[26]

The risk of stroke is 4 to 6 times higher in those with high blood pressure. [4] The prevalence of high blood pressure increases with age and the risk of stroke increases proportionally with increasing blood pressure. [32] High blood pressure is one of the chronic diseases responsible for half of all deaths from heart attacks and cardiac pathologies. In figures, it is the most common neurological disorder worldwide, affecting more than 5% of people over the age of 60. [29]

More than 70% of patients present with systolic blood pressure higher than 140 mmHg and more than 20% above 180 mmHg, which is related to poor prognosis. Weeks prior to haemorrhagic stroke there is an increase in blood pressure compared to patients who develop ischaemic stroke, in which blood pressure is higher than in patients who develop ischaemic stroke.pre-event blood pressure levels are low compared to post ischaemic event blood pressure levels. (33) Poor blood pressure control is the most important population attributable risk factor for cerebrovascular disease, including haemorrhagic (58%) and ischaemic stroke (50%), ischaemic heart disease (55%) and other forms of cerebrovascular disease (58%). [34]

Control of high blood pressure has led to a significant reduction in cases of cerebrovascular disease. Reductions of 10 mm Hg in systolic blood pressure and 5 mm Hg in diastolic blood pressure have been shown to be associated with a 30-40% reduction in the risk of cerebrovascular disease respectively, making adequate blood pressure control one of the main elements in the prevention of new events of transient ischaemic attacks and even ischaemic stroke. [32]

Smoking: Tobacco use is the single largest preventable risk factor globally. It is also a risk factor for 6 of the 8 leading causes of death worldwide, and is responsible for 1 in 6 deaths from non-communicable diseases. The main psychoactive component of tobacco is nicotine, a substance that acts on the central nervous system generating biochemical changes responsible for addiction. [35] Tobacco smoke contains more than 7,000 toxic chemicals, including carbon monoxide, formaldehyde, arsenic and cyanide. These chemicals are transferred from the lungs into the bloodstream, changing and damaging cells throughout the body. The changes caused by these chemicals can increase your risk of stroke. Tobacco use has many effects on the body, including thickening of the blood, increased risk of blood clots and narrowing of the arteries, and restriction of oxygen in the blood. [36] Smoking can contribute by raising blood levels of fibrinogen and other procoagulant substances. [37]

The patient with consumption of 20 cigarettes/day is six times more likely to suffer a stroke compared to a non-smoker. [36] The risk for smokers of <20 cigarettes/day is 3.3% compared to non-smokers, while for smokers of >20 cigarettes/day the risk is 5.66%. [9]

In recent years, the term passive smoking has been coined to describe people who come into contact with smokers and suffer from the harmful effects of tobacco. Typically 15% of the smoke from cigarettes is inhaled by the smoker, while 85% is dispersed in the air; this smoke contains up to three times more nicotine and tar, and five times more carbon monoxide. It has been found that non-smokers exposed to smoke for one hour inhale the equivalent of three cigarettes. [38]

Cigarette smoking is associated with an increased risk for all subtypes of cerebrovascular events. A strong dose-response relationship has been reported for both ischaemic stroke and subarachnoid haemorrhage. [35] The risk of subarachnoid haemorrhage is associated with increased incidence of intracerebral aneurysms in smokers. Smoking may also damage the walls of small cerebral arteries, favouring intraparenchymal haemorrhages. The use of e-cigarettes, due to their nicotine content, is also associated with an increased risk of vascular events, although the risk is probably lower than with conventional cigarette smoking. (39)The relative risk of cerebrovascular disease for smokers is 1.51, being higher for women than for men. [38] The risk of stroke is reduced by quitting smoking. Active smokers have a higher risk of stroke than ex-smokers and this difference is greater in women. It has been estimated that within one year of quitting smoking, the risk of stroke is halved and within five years the risk is equalised. than non-smokers. Smoking cessation as a secondary prevention measure after a stroke or vascular event has also been shown to be beneficial. Dyslipidaemias: Dyslipidaemia is epidemiologically closely associated with vascular diseases. Dyslipidaemias or hyperlipidaemias are metabolic disturbances in blood lipid levels, characterised by increased cholesterol levels as well as increased triglyceride concentrations or also called hypertriglyceridaemia. [39] High triglyceride levels and low HDL-cholesterol (HDL-C) levels are considered risk factors for coronary heart disease and ischaemic stroke. [4]

Many studies have shown its association with atherosclerosis by triggering lipid deposits; biochemical processes that form atherosclerotic plaques inside arterial vessels, which can partially or totally obstruct one or more vessels. These disorders are responsible for a large proportion of cases of acute myocardial infarction and stroke. [40]

The incidence of cerebrovascular disease is related to plasma levels of cholesterol, low-density lipoprotein cholesterol (LDLc), triglycerides and high-density lipoprotein cholesterol (HDLc), especially in individuals over 65 years of age. [41] Several studies show an association between high levels of total cholesterol and LDL cholesterol (LDLc) and increased risk of ischaemic stroke. High triglycerides increase the risk of stroke by 10%. [42]

Alcoholism: There is a clear relationship between heavy alcohol consumption and the risk of stroke. In this case, the relationship between the amount of alcohol consumed and the risk of stroke is not linear, as is the case with smoking. Heavy alcohol consumption is mainly associated with an increased risk of intracerebral haemorrhage. This association may be related to increased blood pressure levels, reduced blood pressure in the brain, and a reduction in the risk of intracerebral haemorrhage. platelet aggregation and increased secretion by endothelial cells of plasminogen activators observed in heavy alcohol consumers. On the other hand, the consumption of large amounts of alcohol in short periods of time is associated with the development of cardiac arrhythmias, including atrial fibrillation, which may be responsible for cardioembolic ischaemic strokes. [39] Alcohol consumption above 60g/day is a risk factor for all types of stroke. However, there seems to be evidence that people who consume less than 24g/day have a lower risk of stroke than abstainers.(4) Physical inactivity and obesity: Physical inactivity has been increasing globally. Most patients who develop a stroke have in common a lack of physical activity and a high level of sedentary pre-stroke lifestyle, marking an association with worse post-stroke outcomes in terms of age at first acute vascular event, degree of motor and neurocognitive dysfunction, as well as stroke recovery and stroke recurrence. People who have had a stroke lead more sedentary lifestyles which may be related to reduced cardio-respiratory fitness, depression, limited mobility, reduced social participation and poor quality of life. [43] There is a significant inverse relationship between physical activity and risk of stroke (ischaemic and haemorrhagic) in both men and women. [9] Obesity, defined as a body mass index (BMI) > 30 kg/m2, is an established risk factor for cardiovascular disease and stroke. [39] Currently, according to the World Health Organisation's International Classification of Diseases, obesity is defined as abnormal or excessive fat storage, secondary to a variety of causes, including energy imbalance, drugs and genetic pathology. [44] Central obesity, measured by waist circumference (> 102 cm in men and > 88 cm in women) is more related to vascular risk than central obesity (> 102 cm in men and > 88 cm in women). overall obesity as measured by BMI 31, and is usually included in the definition of metabolic syndrome. In the INTERSTROKE study, a higher waist-to-hip ratio was significantly associated with the risk of both ischaemic and haemorrhagic stroke.(39) Dietary factors: Diet plays a major role in cerebrovascular health. A healthy diet helps to control and avoid vascular risk factors such as high blood pressure and dyslipidaemia. These dietary interventions can reduce the risk of stroke by up to about 19%. Consumption (Greece - ATTICA study) of cereals, fish and olive oil were associated with low risk of cerebrovascular disease, while sweets, red meat, cheese, margarine, salted nuts, increased the risk. Strokes can be prevented by lowering salt intake and increased consumption of fruit and vegetables, such as wholegrain foods, cereals with fibre and oily fish, confirming these findings on the influence of diet on stroke.(27)Type 2 diabetes mellitus: The role of diabetes mellitus as a risk factor is clearly demonstrated in cerebrovascular disease. [45] Type 2 diabetes mellitus and pre-diabetes are associated with increased vascular risk in parallel with the degree of hyperglycaemia and lack of good metabolic control.[46]There are multiple mechanisms by which diabetes can lead to the development of stroke. These include increased arterial stiffness at an early age, systemic inflammation and capillary membrane thickening, which together lead to subsequent vascular endothelial dysfunction. The function of this endothelial layer is of great importance in maintaining structural integrity as well as vasomotor control. One of the substances that contributes to vasodilation and whose reduced availability could cause endothelial dysfunction and trigger a cascade of atherosclerosis is nitric oxide. For example, vasodilatation mediated by nitric oxide is altered in people with diabetes, possibly due to increased nitric oxide inactivation or decreased smooth muscle reactivity to nitric oxide. People with type II diabetes have stiffer arteries and less elasticity compared to people with normal glucose levels. An increased inflammatory response is often seen in people with diabetes, and inflammation plays an important role in the development of atherosclerotic plaque. C-reactive protein, cytokines and adiponectin are the main serum markers of inflammation. A low level of adiponectin itself has also been associated with stroke. Stroke is two to six times higher in people with diabetes mellitus than in the population without diabetes mellitus. (4) About 60-70% of people who have a stroke have a history of type 2 diabetes mellitus or pre-diabetes 7,8, which in turn are associated with an increased risk of ischaemic recurrence. (46) A diabetic patient, male or female, has a relative risk for any type of cerebrovascular disease ranging from 1.6 to 3. (45,47)It has been shown that the risk of thromboembolic stroke in diabetic men is twice as high as in non-diabetic men, independent of other risk factors. Type 2 diabetics are at higher risk than type 1 diabetics. The coexistence of diabetes and high blood pressure increases the frequency of diabetic complications, including cerebrovascular disease. (47) Early detection, prevention and treatment significantly reduce the development of stroke. Other risk factors, such as obesity and high blood pressure, are often present in people with diabetes, further increasing the risk of stroke. (4)

Atrial fibrillation: Atrial fibrillation is the most common sustained cardiac arrhythmia in humans(48) and is the main embolic cause of ischaemic stroke. (49) It is a supraventricular tachyarrhythmia characterised by disorganised atrial activation with consequent impairment of mechanical function. atrial fibrillation. About 20-30% of all strokes are due to atrial fibrillation. An increasing number of stroke patients are diagnosed with paroxysmal or "silent" atrial fibrillation. The most important complication of atrial fibrillation is cerebral infarction (cerebral embolism). Failure of the atrium to contract effectively can lead to clots in the atrium. If they break off, they can travel through the body's blood vessels. It is responsible for one in six cerebrovascular events. The risk of stroke increases when atrial fibrillation is combined with other risk factors, such as high blood pressure and arteriosclerosis. Atrial fibrillation is not directly associated with haemorrhagic stroke, but haemorrhagic transformation can occur in cerebral infarction. It occurs in 6 % of cases with high mortality. (48)

The pathogenesis of cerebral ischaemia due to atrial fibrillation is based on blood stasis in the left atrium and the consequent formation of thrombi, their detachment and embolism to small arteries in the brain. (49) Therefore, the non-modifiable risk factors or risk markers are: (9) Age: With old age, the individual's functional and cognitive reserve deteriorates. Older age increases the likelihood of cerebrovascular disease, and comorbidities such as hypertension, diabetes, dyslipidaemia and obesity,(8) is well documented that for every decade after the age of 50 the risk of cerebrovascular disease doubles.[1] Age is the major non-modifiable risk factor, the incidence of stroke increases exponentially with age and is highest in people over 65 years of age, which accounts for 7 out of 8 deaths from cerebrovascular disease. It can be argued that the incidence of stroke doubles every decade after the age of 55 years and more than 70% of strokes occur after the age of 65 years. [32]

Gender: Women are disproportionately affected by stroke, both in terms of mortality and morbidity. Clinical evidence from experimental models shows the major role of gonadal hormones, specifically oestrogen is a neuroprotectant, which is why men have more strokes in their youth, but after women enter the menopausal period the risk is much higher in women,[50] this makes women more likely to die from the disease later in life. [5] Stroke in women is evidenced by pre-eclampsia, oral contraceptives, menopause and hormone replacement. Metabolic syndrome, obesity, atrial fibrillation and migraine with aura also contribute as risk factors, so the danger of cerebrovascular ischaemia, both extracranial and intracranial, requires strict control of these factors. Women may have a slightly different clinical presentation profile than men, which causes delayed diagnosis and in turn may lead to delayed treatment, reducing the chance of a favourable prognosis. [2]

One in 5 women will have a stroke, approximately 55,000 more women than men have a stroke each year and it is the fourth leading cause of death in women (over 80,000 women die each year), with black women having the highest prevalence.(27)Hereditary factors: A family history of stroke is associated with an increased risk of stroke. This can be related, on the one hand, to a series of predisposing genetic factors and, on the other, to the sharing of certain environmental, cultural or social factors. [5]

Thrombophilias are the most common inherited disorders associated with cerebrovascular events. Hyperhomocysteinemia is the most frequently associated with these, due to its association with hypercoagulable states. The homocysteine is an essential amino acid derived from methionine metabolism which is metabolised by two pathways: remethylation, in which methionine is recovered from homocysteine with a requirement for vitamin B12, and trans-sulphurisation, which allows the synthesis of cysteine, the elevation of which can lead to neuronal cell damage through toxicity and cause vascular damage, prothrombotic effects and oxidative stress. Cerebral aneurysms are lesions of the arteries that cause weakness and dilatation of a segment of the artery. They usually occur at the bifurcation of the polygon of Wills and their rupture can lead to subarachnoid haemorrhages and thus to severe neurological complications. They have been shown to be autosomal inherited first-degree lesions and have been linked to alterations in the gene encoding nitric oxide synthase, which is expressed in the endothelium and serves as a potent endogenous vasodilator. [24]

Health education.

Primary health care has been presented as a conglomerate of values and principles focused on achieving better health in the population, accessible to all individuals and families in the community, with their full participation and at an affordable cost.

According to the World Health Organisation, health education comprises a set of theoretical-practical learning opportunities with the aim of achieving the development of skills that promote the health of the population[51] , it is the discipline responsible for guiding and organising educational processes with the purpose of positively influencing the knowledge, practices and customs of individuals and communities in relation to their health. It is an area that has seen recent growth in the field, positioning itself as one of the main promotion strategies. [52]

Health Education is currently considered as the educational process to promote and educate on factors that impact on the general population and on each individual. particular individual. It is not just teaching behaviours, but motivating change to create healthy behaviours.

The objective of health education is to make health a collective good, training the population so that they can contribute to their health in a participatory and responsible way, changing harmful behaviours and consolidating healthy ones, therefore, health education is based on Health Promotion and disease prevention, to improve the determinants of health of the entire population and enable the learning of healthy lifestyle habits.

The activities to achieve this have a scientific basis and specific methodologies, techniques and didactic tools to generate an educational process, some of them are through personalised education on an individual basis, or in groups and to cover a greater number of individuals generating educational processes for population groups, some of them are: educational sessions, workshops, guidance, counselling, play activities, self-help groups, among others.(53)

Public health interventions are a set of collective strategies or actions aimed at protecting and promoting health in communities or populations. Each intervention must have a design, an implementation and an evaluation of the results. The results of each intervention are related to multiple social, economic, political, cultural and organisational variables. (51)

Stroke prevention and treatment requires complex interventions to address multiple domains (physiological, psychological, social and environmental) to target human behaviour and the control of vascular risk factors. (54)

Health education and health promotion are closely intertwined, with health education being a tool and a vehicle that, when developed and implemented, can be used to promote health. in conjunction with the active participation of individuals, becomes health promotion. Today, health promotion has become an exercise that involves education, training, research, legislation, policy coordination and community development. (52)

Knowledge, habits and social influence are determinants of health with a high potential for modification; if knowledge is considered to influence attitude leading to changes in health, the strategy would be to develop intervention plans and programmes on risk factors. (55)

Mass action on lifestyle factors is the most cost-effective means of disease prevention. (54)

In this research, an educational intervention was carried out, as it is the process that makes it possible to receive information, produce knowledge on certain health issues and promote reflection. In addition, it stimulates the promotion of healthy habits, prevents illnesses and improves the quality of life, and is a fundamental pillar of health care. It constitutes a suitable resource for achieving changes in lifestyles, mainly at an early age.

METHODOLOGICAL DESIGN

A quasi-experimental intervention study was carried out to assess the impact of an educational programme on cerebrovascular disease risk factors in clinic 11, Manuel Piti Fajardo, Santo Domingo, from January to December 2023. A sample of 35 patients was selected from the population aged 50-60 years dispensed in clinic 11 as being at risk of cerebrovascular disease by non-probability sampling by criteria.

Inclusion criteria:

✓ Having more than 2 risk factors for cerebrovascular disease.

✓ Consent to be part of the research.

Exclusion criteria:

✓ Patients who do not agree to participate.

✓ Patients with mental disabilities.

Data collection methods and techniques.

In order to collect the information, the participants were first explained what the study consisted of and an informed consent form was drawn up for their approval (Appendix 1). Next, a questionnaire was used for this purpose, which was applied to each patient by the author of this research (Appendix 2), where general patient data, history of chronic diseases, toxic habits and a database with the variables of interest were collected.

In addition, a questionnaire (Annex 3) was administered in two parts, Part I to assess knowledge about the types of cerebrovascular disease and Part II to assess knowledge about risk factors for cerebrovascular disease, before and during the study, and Part II to assess knowledge about risk factors for cerebrovascular disease, before and after the study. after the educational programme (Annex 5). Based on the needs identified and the risk factors present in the patients, a programme was designed and implemented after coordination with the participants to establish the most convenient dates and times for its development, which was carried out based on the educational programmes of the speciality theses of Dr. José Silva and Dr. Susana Consuegra, which were adapted according to our objectives, to compare knowledge about types of cerebrovascular disease and risk factors of these diseases, and a grade was given based on the review guide (Appendix 4). In addition, the variation of some risk factors after the educational intervention was evaluated by applying a form (Annex 6) before and after the educational programme, which was filled out by the author of this intervention, where blood pressure was taken and samples were taken to determine the value of glycaemia. The Educational Programme "Stroke in the 21st Century" was made up of 10 activities with a duration of 45 - 90 minutes each session.

Statistical analysis.

The data obtained were recorded in a Microsoft Excel workbook. Subsequently, statistical processing was carried out using SPSS ("Statistical Package for Social Sciences") version 22 for Windows. Analysis techniques were used according to the study design: chi-square and Student's t-test.

Analyses were analysed according to the criterion (Student's t-test): If $p > 0.01$ There is no significant difference before than after. If $p < 0.01$ there is a significant difference before than after. A reliability level of 99 % was set.
Analyses were analysed according to the criterion (chi-square):
If $p > 0.00$ No significant difference before than after If $p < 0.05$ Significant difference before than after.
A reliability level of 95 % was set.
Operationalisation of the variables:

✓ Age: Age in years at the time of the research.
50 - 54 years

55 - 60 years

✓ Sex: according to biological sex of belonging.
Female Male
✓ Risk factors for cerebrovascular disease:

- Ischaemic heart disease: personal pathological history of ischaemic heart disease.
- History of cerebrovascular disease: history of previous cerebrovascular disease.

• Smoking: is the addiction to tobacco, mainly caused by nicotine.
• Diabetes Mellitus
• Arterial Hypertension.

In the case of controllable factors (Diabetes Mellitus and Hypertension) for comparison before and after the intervention were considered according to the criteria:

• Diabetes Mellitus:

Controlled: capillary blood glucose levels 6.1 - 8.8 mmol/l.
Uncontrolled: capillary blood glucose levels more than 10 mmol/l.

• High blood pressure:

Controlled: a patient whose blood pressure has been below 140/90 mmHg in all blood pressure readings over a year (at least 4).

Uncontrolled: a patient whose blood pressure has been less than 60% of 140/90 mmHg or higher over a one-year period.

✓ Knowledge about the types of cerebrovascular diseases.
Adequate: When a score of more than 70 points is obtained in Part I of the cerebrovascular disease questionnaire.

Inadequate: When a score of less than 70 points is obtained in Part I of the cerebrovascular disease questionnaire.

✓ Knowledge about risk factors for cerebrovascular diseases.

Adequate: When a score of more than 70 points is obtained in Part II of the questionnaire on knowledge of cerebrovascular disease risk factors.
Inadequate: When a score of less than 70 points is obtained in Part II of the questionnaire on knowledge of cerebrovascular disease risk factors.

RESULTS

Table 1 showed a predominance of patients in the age group 55 - 60 years with 24 patients representing 68.6 % of the study population, and in terms of sex, the highest percentage was male with 54.3 % of the total. With regard to risk factors (Table 2), it was found that the risk factor with the highest percentage was high blood pressure, with 30 patients (85.7 %). The second most common cause was diabetes mellitus with 18 patients (51.4 %) and smoking with 12 patients (34.3 %). In the case of arterial hypertension, the male sex predominated with 45.7%. Statistically the sex variable is independent of the risk factors, i.e. the risk factors have a similar behaviour for both sexes (p = 0.583).The Educational Programme "Stroke in the 21st century" consisted of 10 activities, with a weekly frequency. Different media were used in its development: banners, blackboard, audiovisuals, leaflets, glucometer. Assessment of knowledge of cerebrovascular disease risk factors before and after implementation of the Educational Programme (Table 3) showed that before the intervention most patients had inadequate knowledge, 27, for 77.1 %. After the Educational Programme was applied, there was an increase in patients' knowledge of the different types of stroke, with 82.8% (29 patients) and only 6 patients had inadequate knowledge (17.1%). These results were highly significant (p = 0.001).In table 4, when comparing the knowledge of risk factors for cerebrovascular disease before and after the intervention, it was observed that before applying the Educational Programme, the majority presented inadequate knowledge (62.8%), and after the intervention, only 4 patients of the total presented inadequate knowledge. represented by 11.4 %, which showed a high increase of information from the patients in this study. With a high statistical significance (p = 0.002) When we analysed table 5 according to patients with controlled and uncontrolled hypertension, it showed that 19 patients had uncontrolled hypertension (54.3 %). After the Educational Programme was applied, only 5 patients were found to have uncontrolled hypertension (14.3 %). These results were highly significant (p = 0.000). According to table 6, before the Educational Programme 23 patients had a smoking habit, which represented 65.7 %, and there was an increase in the number of non-smoking patients after the intervention, 16 patients for 45.7 %. With highly significant results (p = 0.009).When comparing the sample of patients with controlled and uncontrolled Diabetes Mellitus (Table 7), it was found that 10 patients had their underlying disease under control before the Educational Programme was implemented, for 28.6 %. %, with an increase of 45.7 % (16 patients) in controlled patients after applying the Educational Programme. Results with high statistical significance (p= 0.003)

DISCUSSION

In studies carried out on patients diagnosed with cerebrovascular disease in different parts of Cuba, the male sex is the one with the highest incidence of this entity: Piloto Cruz and collaborators[12] find that in the population admitted to the central military hospital from June 2017 to June 2018 with a diagnosis of cerebrovascular disease 58.7% are men; in the Hospital "Comandante Pinares", in the province of Artemisa, between 2016 and 2018, it was found in the intensive therapy service that 56% of patients admitted for cerebrovascular disease were male[16] and in Consolación del sur in a study published by Linares Río M, Pérez López H, Frances Acosta Y, 78% of patients diagnosed with cerebrovascular disease were male[17] , In our results, where we worked with patients at risk of cerebrovascular disease, it is striking that the male population predominated, which coincides with what other authors indicate is the highest incidence of cerebrovascular disease, which is why developing activities to make patients aware of their risk and make them participate in the reduction of these factors is fundamental.Our results were similar to those of the study carried out by Pérez Rodríguez and collaborators[56] during 2018, in the medical office 47 belonging to the Hermanos Cruz de Pinar del Río University Polyclinic, 63.0 % of the sample belonged to the male sex. We agree with Botero Botero and collaborators[8] in a cross-sectional descriptive observational study in older adults with risk factors for cerebrovascular disease in a gerontological centre in Medellín, between 2017-2020, it can be seen that the majority of older adults in this centre are men (51.4%). We disagree with the study carried out by Rico Loaiza and collaborators[22] , in the Nursing Home in the municipality of Caracolí they found that 94.4 % of the women had risk factors for the onset of cerebrovascular disease.In the study by Fuentes González and Pirazán Vergara[6] 57.1 % of patients attending the chronic consultation, Hospital San Antonio de Soatá belong to the female sex and 42.8 % are men. Authors such as Fonte Medina and collaborators[41] in the study in the Clinical Laboratory Service of the General Teaching Hospital "Abel Santamaría Cuadrado" Pinar del Río, during the period 2013 - 2014 there is a large predominance of women 61 % with more than two risk factors for cerebrovascular disease compared to men. According to the literature, arterial hypertension is the most important risk factor for both cerebral ischaemia and cerebral haemorrhage; it is the trigger for cerebrovascular disease in 75% of cases, and is therefore the most common and the most important[47] . Our results are in agreement with Córdova López[55] in their study, Arterial Hypertension with 75.00 % and Diabetes Mellitus (73.50

%). %) in that order constitute the predominant risk factors for the development of cerebrovascular disease.We agree with the study by Fuentes González and Pirazán Vergara[6] in patients attending the chronic consultation, Hospital San Antonio de Soatá, the most relevant pathology is arterial hypertension, present in 10 interviewees, which corresponds to 71.4%. Botero Botero[8] , in his study between 2017-2020 on risk factors for cerebrovascular disease in a gerontological centre in Medellín shows that the most representative risk factors for suffering a stroke are BMI >= 25 with 75.7%.%, followed by high blood pressure (67.6 %) and no physical activity (48.6 %). Dr. Pérez Rodríguez and collaborators[56] , in their research, point out sedentary lifestyles (61.5%), high blood pressure (44.6%), smoking (23%) in that order. In our results, we found some points in common regarding the risk factors indicated by these authors, but we differed in their frequency, as hypertension predominated and in a higher percentage than those found in these two populations.Once the educational programme was implemented, there was an increase in knowledge about the risk factors for cerebrovascular diseases, a result that coincides with that of Córdova López[55] in Cuenca, Ecuador, 38.64% of the participants before the intervention did not recognise that diseases such as Diabetes Mellitus and Arterial Hypertension are risk factors for stroke, after the educational intervention this percentage was reduced to 16%. The educational programme not only increased knowledge about the types of cerebrovascular diseases and their risk factors, but also motivated a change in behaviour favourable to the control of hypertension and diabetes mellitus.The application of the Educational Programme in Clinic 11, Manuel Piti Fajardo Polyclinic, in the patients in the sample, increased their knowledge of the different types of cerebrovascular disease and its risk factors and modified their behaviour in favour of better health education. The intervention achieved a significant positive change in the behaviour of risk factors for developing cerebrovascular disease in the patients, such as: Arterial Hypertension, Diabetes Mellitus and smoking.After its implementation, the Educational Programme had a positive influence on the knowledge, practices and habits of the patients in the study in relation to their health. At the same time, it enabled the population to learn healthy lifestyle habits. Having two or three risk factors means that a person is more likely to suffer a stroke, so prevention is of vital importance. In more than 90 % of patients diagnosed with acute stroke are found to have two or more atherogenic risk factors, which, whether or not associated with chronic non-communicable diseases, play an important role in the short-, medium- and long-term prognosis of the disease. The identification of non-modifiable risk factors is important because, although it is not possible to take measures for their elimination or modification, they help to identify individuals at increased risk for stroke. [56] In the author's opinion, the change in controllable risk factors for cerebrovascular disease, hypertension and diabetes mellitus, as well as a slight decrease in the number of smokers, indicates that raising awareness and involving patients in the health-disease process, generating positive and healthy behaviours, can influence risk factors and in turn influence future illness.

CONCLUSIONS

In the population between 50 and 60 years of age, who are classified as being at risk of cerebrovascular disease in clinic 11, men predominate and high blood pressure, diabetes mellitus and smoking are the factors that stand out in that order. The application of the Educational Programme has had a favourable impact, since after its implementation, favourable changes in health have been observed both in the knowledge and behaviour of the population regarding the control and reduction of risk factors.

RECOMMENDATIONS

- The author recommends the application of this Educational Programme in the other clinics of the Manuel Piti Fajardo Polyclinic, as well as its extension to other health centres.

REFERENCES

1. Rivera Ramirez F, Duarte Troche MC, Tenorio Borroto E, Orozco González CN. Risk factors for stroke in young adults. Rev. de Ciencias de la Salud 2020 vol.7 no.22 1-11.Available at : https://www.ecorfan.org/bolivia/researchjournals/Ciencias_de_la_Salud/vol7num22/Revista_Ciencias_de_la_Salud_V7_N22_1.pdf

2. Rojas N, Carbó Cisnero Y, León Guilart A. Risk factors associated with cerebrovascular disease in women. Rev. Cubana de Medicina [Internet]. 2022 [cited 20 Feb 2024]; 61 (1) Available from: https://revmedicina.sld.cu/index.php/med/article/view/2542

3. Pérez Guerra LE, Rodríguez Flores O, López García ME, Sánchez Fernández M, Alfonso Arboláez LE, Monteagudo Méndez Cruz I. Knowledge of stroke and its risk factors in older adults. Acta med centre [Internet]. 2022 Mar [cited 2023 Aug 20]; 16(1): 69-78. Available from: http://scielo.sld.cu/scielo.php?script=sci_arttext&pid=S2709792720220001000 69&lng=en. Epub 31-Mar-2022.

4. Correa Villalón FA. Description of risk factors associated with ischemic stroke in patients attended in the medical service of the Regional Hospital of Huacho. Thesis for the degree of surgeon. School of Human Medicine;2022. Available at : https://repositorio.unjfsc.edu.pe/handle/20.500.14067/6445

5. Valdivielso Gómez L. "Código ictus": Atención urgente. Final degree thesis. Faculty of Nursing. University of Cantabria;2020. Available at : https://repositorio.unican.es/xmlui/bitstream/handle/10902/20085/

6. Fuentes Gonzalez N, Pirazán Vergara AV. Perception of stroke in patients with chronic noncommunicable diseases. 2022;19(3):86-95 .Available at :https://doi.org/10.22463/17949831.3477

7. Gutiérrez López Y- leen, Chang Fonseca D, Carranza Zamora AJ. Acute ischemic cerebrovascular event. Rev. med. sinerg. [Internet]. May 1, 2020 [cited April 28, 2024];5(5): e476. Available from: https://revistamedicasinergia.com/index.php/rms/article/view/476

8. Botero Botero LM, Pérez Pérez JM, Duque Vázquez DA, Quintero Reyes CA. Risk factors for cerebrovascular disease in the elderly. Rev Cubana Med Gen Integr. 2021;37(3):1-16. Available at: www.medigraphic.com/cgi-

bin/new/resumen.cgi?IDARTICULO=110067

9. Pérez Rodríguez MA. Knowledge about Stroke in the population of Santa Cruz de La Palma: University of La Laguna; 2017-2018. Final Degree Thesis. Sede La Palma. 2017-2018.

10. Topacio Rodríguez MA, Ortiz Galeano I. Clinical characteristics of patients with ischemic stroke admitted during the therapeutic window period in the Emergency Department of the Hospital de Clínicas. An. Fac. Cienc. Méd. (Asunción), August - 2022; 55(2): 18-24.

11. Molina Ramírez Y, Díaz Chalala JE, Yera Jaramillo BL, Bolufé Vilaza ME, Núñez Mora S. Behaviour of acute cerebrovascular disease in a rural area. Rev. inf. sci. [Internet]. 2021 Aug [cited 2023 Aug 20]; 100(4): e3484. Available from: http://scielo.sld.cu/scielo.php?script=sci_arttext&pid=S1028-99332021000400011&lng=en. Epub 24-Jun-2021.

12. Piloto Cruz A, Suarez Rivero B, Belaunde Clausell A, Castro JM. Cerebrovascular disease and its risk factors. Rev Cub Med Mil [Internet]. 2020 Sep [cited 2023 Aug 20]; 49(3): e568.Available from: http://scielo.sld.cu/scielo.php?script=sci_arttext&pid=S0138-65572020000300009&lng=en. Epub 25-Nov-2020

13. Calderón Sanginez J, Abanto Argomedo CS, Otiniano Sifuentes DR, Berrú Villalobos SE, Chong Chinchay K, Reyes E, Pozzi Angulo MF. Epidemiological Bulletin. National Institute of Neurological Sciences. No. 1.2022 Available at: https://www.gob.pe/institucion/instituto-nacional-de-ciencias-neurologicas/informes-publicaciones/562151515-boletin-epidemiologico-n-01-2022-incn

14. Soto Á, Guillén Grima F, Morales G, Muñoz S, Aguinaga-Ontoso I, Fuentes-Aspe R. Prevalence and incidence of stroke in Europe: systematic review and meta-analysis. Anales Sis San Navarra [Internet]. 2022 Apr [cited 2024 Apr 29]; 45(1): e0979. Available from: http://scielo.isciii.es/scielo.php?script=sci_arttext&pid=S1137-66272022000100012&lng=en.Epub 07-Nov 2022. https://dx.doi.org/10.23938/assn.0979.

15. Gamarra Insfrán JL, Soares Sanches R, Fernandes Sanches CJ. Risk factors associated with ischemic stroke in patients attended in a public hospital in Paraguay. Rev. Inst. Med. Trop. [Internet]. Dec. 2020 [cited 2023 Aug 20]; 15(2): 45-52. Available from: http://scielo.iics.una.py/scielo.php?script=sci_arttext&pid=S1996-

36962020000200045&lng=en. https://doi.org/10.18004/imt/2020.15.2.45.

16. Moreira Diaz LR, Torres Ordaz A, Peña Rodriguez A, Palenzuela Ramos Y. Cerebrovascular disease in patients admitted to intensive care. Rev Medical Sciences [Internet]. 2020 [cited: Date of access].24(4):e4316.Available from: http://revcmpinar.sld.cu/index.php/publicaciones/article/view/4316

17. Linares-Río M, Pérez-López H, Frances-Acosta Y. Characterization of risk factors for cerebrovascular disease in people over 60 years of age. Revista Cubana de Medicina [Internet]. 2022 [cited 28 Apr 2024];61(3) Available at: https://revmedicina.sld.cu/index.php/med/article/view/2490

18. Health Statistical Yearbook 2020. Ministry of Public Health. Direccion de Registros Médicos y Estadisticas de Salud. Havana:MINSAP; 2020 (Cited 2021).Internet:https://temas.sld.cu/estadisticassalud/ http://bvscuba.sld.cu/anuario-estadistico-de-cuba/

19. Agarica Aguilar Y, Curbelo Lopez M. Prognostic value of glycemia in the neurological evolution of diabetic patients with cerebrovascular disease. Rev. Cuban de Med [Internet]. Dec 2022 [cited 2024 Feb 21]; 61(4): e2708. Available from: http://scielo.sld.cu/scielo.php?script=sci_arttext&pid=S0034-75232022000400005&lng=en. Epub 01-Dec-2022.

20. Ruiz Mariño RA, Campos Muñoz M, Rodríguez Campos D, Chacón Reyes OD. Clinical and tomographic characteristics of patients with ischaemic cerebrovascular disease. MEDISAN [Internet]. 2021 Jun [cited 2024 Apr 28]; 25(3): 624-636. Available from: http://scielo.sld.cu/scielo.php?script=sci_arttext&pid=S1029-30192021000300624&lng=en. Epub 04-Jun-2021.

21. García-Alfonso C, Martínez Reyes A,García V, Ricaurte-Fajardo A, Torres I, Coral J. Update on diagnosis and treatment of acute ischemic stroke. Univ. Med.2019;60(3). https://doi.org/10.11144/Javeriana.umed 60-3.actu

22. Rico Loaiza A, Trujillo Puerta JP, Castrillon López ND, Arango Parra V, Posada Quintero W. Knowledge in the early detection of an accident. cerebrovascular by the community at risk in the municipality of Caracolí. Degree work. Faculty of Medicine. Medellín. 2020.

23. Borja Santillán, M. A., Samaniego Gallino, J. L., Aguirre Ruilova, S. D.,Prieto Ulloa, M. G. (2021). Ischemic cerebrovascular disease and arterial hypertension in the Teodoro Maldonado Carbo Hospital. RECIMUNDO,5(Especial1),31-

42. Available at :https://doi.org/10.26820/recimundo/5.(esp.1).nov.2021.31-42
24. Conde-Cardona G, Medrano-Carreazo JC, Parada-Artunduaga MD, et al. Cerebrovascular disease in young patients: key aspects of the literature. Acta Neurol Colomb. 2021; 37(1): 39-48. Available at: https://doi.org/10.22379/24224022361

25. Nuñez Morales AM, Sanchez A. Predictive Analysis of Cerebrovascular Accidents in Patients aged 18-65 years of the Preventive Health Control Program with artificial intelligence (CSPia) with Selvy Checkup technology in the Period 2019-2020 in the National Institute for Research of Infectious-Contagious Diseases (INIEICONT) Santo Domingo, Dominican Republic. Preliminary Final Project to opt for the degree of Doctor of Medicine. Santo Domingo, National District. June 2021. Available at : https://repositorio.unibe.edu.do/jspui/handle/123456789/585

26. Noya Chaveco ME, Moya González NL, Llamos Sierra N, Morales Larramendi R, Cardona Garbey DL, Filiú Ferrera JL, et al. Temas de Medicina Interna. 5 -ed. Havana: Editorial Ciencias Médicas, 2017.

27. Rojas Daza JD, Salles Rojas MC. Risk factors associated with stroke in adult and elderly patients attended in the emergency department of the Regional Hospital of Pucallpa. Thesis to opt for the title of second specialty in interdisciplinary. Peru. 2022.

28. Psyciencia. Cerebrovascular Accident (CVA): definition, types and treatment [Internet]. Psyciencia editorial team. 2019. Available from:https://www.psyciencia.com/accidente-cerebrovascular-acv- definition-types-and-treatment/

29. Martínez-Cáceres MJ, Rubio-Duarte MC, Zambrano-Medina NA, Llanos-Redondo A, Pérez-Reyes GV, Rangel-Navia HJ.Rev Latinoamericana de Hipertensión.Vol.17.Nº2,2022. Available at: https://www.revhipertension.com/rlh_2_2022/10_hipertension_arterial_factor.pdf

30. Torres Pérez RF, Quinteros León MS, Pérez Rodríguez MR, Molina Toca EP, Ávila Orellana FM, Molina Toca SF,et al. Risk factors for essential hypertension and cardiovascular risk. Rev Latinoamericana de Hipertensión. Vol. 16. Nº 4, 2021. Available at: https://www.revhipertension.com/rlh_4_2021/9_factores_riesgo_hipertensio_arterial.pdf

31. Choreño-Parra JA, Carnalla-Cortés M,Guadarrama-Ortíz P. Ischemic

cerebral vascular disease: extensive review of the literature for the first-contact physician. Med Int Mexico. 2019 Jan-Feb;35(1):61-79.https://doi.org/10.24245/mim. v35i1.2212
32. Bender-del-Busto J. Cerebrovascular diseases as a health problem. Revista Cubana de Neurología y Neurocirugía [journal on the Internet]. 2019 [cited 2024 Aug 8]; 9(2): [approx. 0 p.]. Available from: https://revneuro.sld.cu/index.php/neu/article/view/335

33. Viruez Soto A, Chambi Quilla G, Chambi Quilla A, Quispe Ticona N, Jiris Quinteros J, Vera Carrasco O. Stroke in intensive care at very high altitude. Rev. Méd. La Paz [Internet]. 2023 [cited 2024 Aug 08]; 29(2): 30-37. Available from: http://www.scielo.org.bo/scielo.php?script=sci_arttext&pid=S1726-89582023000200030&lng=es. Epub 30-Dec-2023.

34. Martinez R, Soliz P, Campbell NRC, Lackland DT, Whelton PK, Ordunez P. Association between population hypertension and ischaemic heart disease control and stroke mortality in 36 countries and territories of the Americas,1990-2019: an ecological study. Rev Panam Salud Publica. 2023;47:e124. https://doi.org/10.26633/RPSP.2023.124.

35. Reyes-Méndez C, Fierros-Rodríguez C, Cárdenas-Ledesma R, Hernández-Pérez A, García-Gómez L, Pérez-Padilla R. Cardiovascular effects of smoking. Neumol. cir. thorax [journal on the Internet]. 2019 Mar [cited 2024 Aug 08]; 78(1): 56-62. Available from: http://www.scielo.org.mx/scielo.php?script=sci_arttext&pid=S0028-37462019000100056&lng=en. Epub 09-Nov-2020.

36. Gutierrez Baños JJ. Smoking and Stroke. [Internet]2020. Available at: https://es.linkedin.com/pulse/cigarrillo-y-stroke-josé-gutierréz

37. Matamoros Cuadra PI. Prognosis of ischemic cerebrovascular disease according to risk factors January-November 2018. Monograph for the title of specialist in Internal Medicine. Managua, Nicaragua. National Autonomous University of Nicaragua; 2019. Available at : https://repositorio.unan.edu.ni/11288/1/100403.pdf

38. Matías-Pérez D, Pérez-Campos E, García-Montalvo IA. A genetic view of familial hypercholesterolemia. Nutr. Hosp. [Internet]. 2015 Dec [cited 2022 Dec 12]; 32(6): 2421-2426. Available from: http://dx.doi.org/10.3305/nh.2015.32.6.9885.

39. García Pastor A, Cancio Martínez E, Rodríguez Yañez M, Alonso de

Leciñana M, Amaro S, Arenillas JF, et al. Recommendations of the Sociedad Española de Neurology for stroke prevention. Action on lifestyle habits and atmospheric pollution. Neurology 36 (2021) 377-387. Available at : https://www.elsevier.es/es-revista-neurologia-295-articulo-recomendaciones-sociedad-espanola-neurologia-prevencion-S0213485320302280

40. Rivero Truit FA, Pérez Rivero V. Educational intervention for the prevention of complications in patients with dyslipidemia. Rev. Med. Electron. [Internet]. 2019 Dec [cited 2024 Mar 29]; 41(6): 1354-1366. Available from: http://scielo.sld.cu/scielo.php?script=sci_arttext&pid=S1684-18242019000601354&lng=en. Epub 31-Dec-2019.

41. Fonte Medina NC, Llanes Lobo J, Bencomo Fonte LM, Pérez Álvarez Y, Fonseca Medina Y. Atherogenic markers and metabolic syndrome in the urban population of older adults in Pinar del Río. Rev Medical Sciences [Internet]. 2019 Feb [cited 2024 Mar 29]; 23(1): 79-89. Available from: http://scielo.sld.cu/scielo.php?script=sci_arttext&pid=S1561-31942019000100079&lng=en.

42. Palacio Portilla EJ, Roquer J, Amaro S, Arenillas JF, Ayo Martín O, Castellanos M , et al . Dyslipidemias and stroke prevention: recommendations of the Cerebrovascular Diseases Study Group of the Spanish Society of Neurology. Neurología 37 (2022) 61-72. Available at: https://www.elsevier.es/es-revista-neurologia-295-avance-resumen-dislipidemias- prevencion-del-ictus-recomendaciones-S0213485320302991.

43. Gómez Maldonado JG, Chavez Díaz MF, Silva Cañavera SM, Velandia Fonseca HA, Dussán Gorzón D et al.Sedentarismo amenaza silente en el accidente cerebrovascular isquémico-ACV. Scientific & Education Medical Journal.Vol.8,N°2,2022. Available at : https://www.medicaljournal.com.co/index.php/mj/article/download/110/209/553

44. Aguilera C, Labbé T, Busquets J, Venegas P, Neira C, Valenzuela A. Obesity: Risk factor or disease? Rev. med. chile [Internet]. 2019 Apr [cited 2024 Apr 26]; 147(4): 470-474. Disponible en: http://www.scielo.cl/scielo.php?script=sci_arttext&pid=S0034-98872019000400470&lng=es. http://dx.doi.org/10.4067/S0034-98872019000400470.

45. Angarica-Aguilar Y, Salazar-Rodríguez J, Herrera-Arrebato D, Despaigne-Carrión E, Hechevarría-Heredia M, Reina-Rodríguez C. Characterization of ischemic cerebrovascular disease in diabetic patients at the Hospital

Universitario Clínico Quirúrgico General Calixto García. Revista Finlay [journal on the Internet]. 2023 [cited 2024 Feb 20]; 13(3):[approx. 8 p.]. Available from: https://revfinlay.sld.cu/index.php/finlay/article/view/1265

46. Fuentes B, Amaro S, Alonso de Leciñana M, et al. Stroke prevention in patients with type 2 diabetes mellitus or prediabetes. Recommendations of the Cerebrovascular Diseases Study Group of the Spanish Society of Neurology. Neurologia. 2021 May;36(4):305-323. Available at:www.elsevier.es/Neurologia

47. González Gutiérrez CA, Melgara Canales A, Ferrufino Zamora C. Predominant risk factors in Cerebrovascular Disease in patients admitted to the Internal Medicine ward of the Victoria Motta-Jinotega Hospital from January 2016 to June 2016. Thesis for the degree of medical surgeon. Multidisciplinary Regional Faculty, UNAN CUR- MATAGALPA, 2019. Available at : https://repositorio.unan.edu.ni/11257/

48. Ochoa Reina E, Pastrana Márquez Y. Atrial fibrillation and ischemic stroke. Revista Cubana de Medicina Física y Rehabilitación 2020;12(1):e411. Available at: https://www.medigraphic.com/pdfs/revcubmedfisreah/cfr-2020/cfr201g.pdf

49. Cruz Peña E, Arribas Pérez C, Domínguez Guerra LM, José Rodríguez A. Clinical epidemiological behaviour of cerebral infarction in patients with atrial fibrillation. Progaleno Journal Vol 2(2)2019. Available at : http://www.revprogaleno.sld.cu/

50. Duarte J, Lobo R, Rhenals S, Ruiz J. Trends in stroke mortality in the Department of Atlántico: 1985 to 2014. Thesis. Universidad del Norte. Barranquilla. 2020. Available at : https://manglar.uninorte.edu.co/handle/10584/9731

51. Sánchez Duque JA, Soto Vásquez JP, Cuadrado Guevara RA, Gómez González JF, Rodríguez Morales AJ. Strategies for Community Health Intervention in a Multidisciplinary University Research and Service Camp. Rev Cubana Med Gen Integr [Internet]. 2019 Sep [cited 2024 Aug 22]; 35(3): Available from: http://scielo.sld.cu/scielo.php?script=sci_arttext&pid=S0864212520190003000005&lng=en. Epub 01-Sep-2019

52. Hernández Sarmiento JM, Jaramillo Jaramillo LI, Villegas Alzate JD, Álvarez Hernández LF, Roldan Tabares MD, Ruiz Mejía C, et al. Health education as an important promotion and prevention strategy. Archivos de Medicina (Col), vol. 20, no. 2, pp. 490-504, 2020. Available at:

https://revistasum.umanizales.edu.co/ojs/index.php/archivosmedicina/article/view/3487
53. Guardia Gutiérrez MA, Ruvalcaba Ledezma JC. Health and its determinants, health promotion and health education. Journal of Negative and No Positive Results, vol. 5, no. 1, pp. 81-90, 2020. Available at : https://www.redalyc.org/journal/5645/564563417005/html/

54. Meza Miranda ER, Romero Espínola NR, Báez Ortíz EA. Modifiable risk factors for cerebrovascular disease in stroke patients. Rev. Nutr. Clin. Metab. 2021;4(4):24-31. Available at: https://revistanutricionclinicametabolismo.org/index.php/nutricionclinicametabolismo/article/view/317/556

55. Córdova López PF. Experimental study of educational intervention in knowledge, attitudes and practices for stroke. Rev de la Facultad de Ciencias Médicas Universidad de Cuenca.Vol. 37 Núm.3(2019) Available at : https://publicaciones.ucuenca.edu.ec/ojs/index.php/medicina/article/view/2733

56. Pérez Rodríguez J, Álvarez Velázquez LL, Islas Hernández H, Rivera Alonso E. Risk factors for cerebrovascular disease in older adults in a family medical practice. Rev Medical Sciences [Internet]. 2019 [cited: date accessed]; 23(6): 949-956. Available from: http://revcmpinar.sld.cu/index.php/publicaciones/article/view/4072

ANNEXES

Annex 1. Individual questionnaire.

- Name and surname:

- Age:

- Sex:

- Risk factors. Mark with an X:

Arterial Hypertension

Diabetes Mellitus

Ischaemic heart disease

History of cerebrovascular disease

Smoking

Annex 2. Knowledge questionnaire.

Name and surname:
Age:

Sex:

Part I. Knowledge about cerebrovascular disease.

1. Fill in the blanks:

Stroke refers to any condition in which an area of the brain is affected by ischaemia or haemorrhage. by ischaemia or haemorrhage.

Cerebrovascular disease is the leading cause of cause of death.

The risk factors for cerebrovascular diseases are classified as follows

2. Bookmark with a X which you consider that are cerebrovascular diseases:

Cerebral infarction.

Intraparenchymal haemorrhage. Migraine.
Asymptomatic.

Head trauma.

Vascular dementia.

Subarachnoid haemorrhage. Diabetic neuropathy.
Hypertensive encephalopathy. Transient ischaemic attack.

Part II. Knowledge about risk factors for cerebrovascular disease.

1. Mark with an x those that you consider to be risk factors for cerebrovascular disease:

Smoking. Daily coffee consumption. High blood pressure.
Diabetes Mellitus. Adolescence.

Ischaemic heart disease.

History of cerebrovascular disease. Low blood cholesterol levels.
Use of contraceptive tablets. Systematic physical exercise.

2. Mark T or F:

Having risk factors influences the development of cerebrovascular diseases.

Control of diabetes mellitus is crucial to prevent cerebrovascular disease.

The hypertension hypertension decompensated no trigger a cerebrovascular disease.

3. Tick T or F

There is no link between cerebrovascular disease and diabetes mellitus.

Smoking is a major risk factor for the development of these diseases.

Cerebrovascular disease is more common in younger people.

Submit several factors of risk factors increases the risk of cerebrovascular diseases.
A style of lifestyle prevents the onset of cerebrovascular diseases.

Annex 3. Guide to review of the knowledge questionnaire applied to patients

Name and surname:

Age:

Sex:

Part I. Knowledge about cerebrovascular disease.

1. Fill in the blanks:

Stroke refers to any condition in which an area of the brain is temporarily or permanently affected by ischaemia or haemorrhage.

Cerebrovascular disease is the third leading cause of death.

Factors of risk of cerebrovascular diseases cerebrovascular diseases are classified modifiable or non-modifiable.

Value: 40 points. For correct completion of the 5 options 40 points, 4 correct 35 points points, 3 correct 30 points, 2 correct 25 points, 1 correct 20 points.

2. Bookmark with a X which you considerthat are cerebrovascular diseases:

Cerebral infarction.

X Intraparenchymal haemorrhage.

Migraine.

X Asymptomatic.

Head trauma.

X Vascular dementia.

X Subarachnoid haemorrhage.

Diabetic neuropathy.

Headache

X Hypertensive encephalopathy.

X Transient ischaemic attack.

Value: 60 points. For marking the 6 correct 60 points, 5 correct 55 points, 4 correct 55 points, 4 correct 55 points, 4 correct 55 points, 4 correct 55 points, 4 correct 55 points, 4 correct 55 points.

correct 50 points, 3 correct 45 points, 2 correct 40 points and 1 correct 35 points. For marking an incorrect one, 1 point is deducted.

The total sum of the questions is 100 points. A patient who scores at least 70 points out of the total number of points shall be considered to have passed the questionnaire.

Adequate level of knowledge: When a score of more than 70 points is obtained.

Inadequate level of knowledge: When a score of less than 70 points is obtained.

Part II. Knowledge about risk factors for cerebrovascular disease.

1. Mark with an x those that you consider to be risk factors for cerebrovascular disease:

X Smoking.

Daily coffee consumption. X High blood pressure.
X Diabetes Mellitus.

Adolescence.
X Ischaemic heart disease.
X History of cerebrovascular disease.

X Low blood cholesterol levels. X Use of contraceptive pills.
Systematic practice of physical exercise.

Value: 50 points. For scoring the 6 correct 50 points, 5 correct 45 points, 4 correct 45 points, 4 correct 45 points, 4 correct 50 points.

correct 40 points, 3 correct 35 points, 2 correct 30 points and 1 correct 25 points.

For marking an incorrect one, 1 point is deducted.

2. Mark T or F:

VPresent factors from risk factors influences a that occurrence of cerebrovascular diseases.

Control of diabetes mellitus is crucial to prevent cerebrovascular disease.

FDecompensated hypertension does not trigger cerebrovascular disease.

Value: 25 points. For 2 true 15 points, for each one 7.5 points. For the false one 10 points.

3. Tick T or F

F There is no relationship between cerebrovascular disease and diabetes mellitus.

Smoking is a major risk factor for the development of these diseases.

F Cerebrovascular disease is more common in younger people.

Having several risk factors increases the risk of cerebrovascular disease.

VUn style from lifestyle prevents the onset of cerebrovascular diseases.

Value: 25 points. For 3 true 15 points, 5 points each. For 2 phalluses 10 points, 5 points each.

The total sum of the questions is 100 points. A patient who scores at least 70 points out of the total number of points shall be considered to have passed the questionnaire.

Adequate level of knowledge: When a score of more than 70 points is obtained.

Inadequate level of knowledge: When a score of less than 70 points is obtained.

Annex 4 . Educational Programme

"Stroke in the 21st century".

Activity 1.

Theme: Time to get to know each other.

Summary: Presentation of each of the patients in the study.

Objectives: To get patients to get to know each other and achieve bonding in the group.

Time: 30 minutes.

Method: Conversation.

Means: Cards.

Responsible: Principal Investigator.

Participatory technique used: By cards.

Procedure: Each of the patients in the group puts their name and some identifying characteristics of themselves on a card and shows it to the rest of the group. This should be done for everyone.

Activity 2.

Topic: General overview of cerebrovascular disease.

Contents:

- Behaviour of cerebrovascular diseases in Cuba and in the world.
- Causes and types of cerebrovascular diseases.
- Main symptoms of cerebrovascular diseases.

Objectives:

• To learn about the behaviour of cerebrovascular diseases in Cuba and the world.

• To know the causes and types of cerebrovascular diseases.

• Recognise the main symptoms of cerebrovascular diseases.

Time: 90 minutes.

Method: Expository - Illustrative.

Media: Blackboard, audiovisuals.

Responsible: Principal Investigator.

Participatory technique used: Questions and answers.

Procedure: A brief presentation will be given on how cerebrovascular diseases behave in Cuba and in the world, followed by questions and answers on the different types and causes of cerebrovascular diseases, as well as some of the symptoms that may occur.

Activity 3.

Theme: Myths and facts about cerebrovascular diseases.

Contents:

• Are cerebrovascular diseases hereditary?

• Is it true that if I have already had a stroke, can I have another one?

• Are they preventable?

Objectives:

• To know whether cerebrovascular diseases are hereditary.

• Determine whether a patient who has had a stroke episode is likely to have another one.

• To know whether cerebrovascular diseases are preventable.

Time: 45 minutes

Method: Expository - Illustrative.

Media: Foldables, audiovisuals.

Responsible: Principal Investigator.

Participatory technique employed (At the beginning of the activity): Myths and realities.

Materials required: None.

Procedure: Two spaces will be established in the classroom, one "Myths" and the other "Myths". Reality" and explain to the participants that a myth is a false belief that is passed on to each generation and reality is what is true. Related sentences will be read out on the topic and each participant will go to the space in the classroom that corresponds to him/her. Each participant must explain the reason for their choice. This will be done in a dynamic way.

Activity 4.

Theme: General on the factors of risk factors from the cerebrovascular diseases.

Contents:

• Risk factors for cerebrovascular disease that can be modified.

• Risk factors for cerebrovascular disease that cannot be modified.

Objectives:

• Know the risk factors for cerebrovascular disease that can be modified.

• Know the risk factors for cerebrovascular disease that cannot be modified.

• Describe the risk factors for cerebrovascular diseases.

Time: 90 minutes
Method: Joint elaboration.

Media: Foldables, audiovisuals.

Responsible: Principal Investigator.

Participatory technique used (At the beginning of the activity): Brainstorming.

Materials required: None.

Procedure: the "Brainstorming" reflection technique is applied to carry out the debate on the topic to be worked on. At the end of the participatory technique, the facilitator of the activity will explain in clear language the main risk factors of cerebrovascular diseases and which are modifiable or not.

Activity 5.

Theme: I practice and exercise how to measure blood pressure.

Objectives: To clarify the algorithm and requirements for blood pressure measurement.

Duration: 2 hours.

Via: Reflective Workshops.

Methods: Discussion.
Procedures: Explanation, analysis and synthesis.

Technique: Questions and answers.

Media: Cardboard banners, flipchart and office supplies.
Activities:

Introduction: The session will start by recalling aspects of the previous meeting on_ the procedure for the practice and the exercise on how to measure AT.

Main activity

First moment.

In this activity, the presence of the nurses and doctors from the clinic is of great importance, as they will be responsible for developing the activity together with the researcher. It is proposed to divide the group of patients randomly into two subgroups: A and B. In each of them there should be representatives of all ages, over 19 years of age. Group A: Evaluators (One doctor and one nurse) Group B: Evaluees (One doctor and one nurse) Each group will be evaluated by taking blood pressure samples in the selected patients, using the paper-and-opponent technique. Each group leader will fill in a form taking into account the following classification:

Classification of blood pressure according to adult figures: Blood Pressure (systolic BP) (mmHg) Normal to 120 Blood Pressure (diastolic BP) (mmHg) to 80 High Blood Pressure 130 or more than 85. Based on the average of two or more readings taken at each of two or more readings after the initial screening. When systolic or diastolic blood pressure figures fall into different categories, the highest of the pressures is the one taken to assign the classification category.

By blood pressure number:

SYSTEMIC TA DIASTOLIC TA DIASTOLIC Light 140 - 159 90 - 99
Moderate 160 - 179 100 - 109
Severe 180 - 210 110 - 119

Very severe > 210 > 120

In a second part of the activity, there will be a dance therapy.

Closure: At the end of the activity, a discussion on patients' lifestyles will be established and patients will be asked to summarise on a flipchart the main ideas to promote healthy lifestyles.

Activity 6.

Theme: I practice and exercise how to measure blood glucose.

Objectives:

1. Prisar el algoritmo y requisitos para realizar la medición de la glucemia.
Duration: 2 hours. Via: Reflective workshops.

Methods: Joint elaboration. Procedures: Explanation, analysis and synthesis. Technique: Questions and answers, thought-provoking drawings. Media: Cardboard banners, glucometer and office supplies. Activities:
Introduction: The session will begin with a discussion of cerebrovascular disease and its risk factors.

Main activity.

In this activity, the presence of the specialists or technicians from the clinical laboratory is of great importance, as they will be responsible, together with the researcher, for carrying out the activity.

The methodology and requirements for proper capillary blood glucose measurement using the Suma portable glucometer are explained, followed by the execution of the test.

Once the blood glucose measurement is completed, participants are invited to find their partner, hold hands and perform 10 squats.
Closing: The session will end with the participatory technique "Drawings to generate reflection", evaluating and reinforcing the knowledge imparted.

Activity 7.

Theme: "Stop smoking for you and your family".
Contents:

- Damages of smoking to your and your family's health.

- Where to go if I want to quit smoking?

- What influence does smoking have on cerebrovascular disease?

- General advice on how to stop smoking. Objectives:
- Identify the harms of smoking to you and your family's health.

- Know where to go to quit smoking.

- Meet at which influences the habit of smoking at the cerebrovascular diseases.

- Demonstrate general tips for smoking cessation. Time: 90 minutes

Method: Expository - Illustrative.

Media: banner and blackboard.

Responsible: Principal Investigator and GBT Psychologist.

Participative technique used: Crossword puzzle.

Materials required: None.

Procedure: In this activity, the crossword technique will be applied, which consists of filling in the spaces of a crossword puzzle previously placed on the blackboard, where the key word is "damage". Each of the participants will go on to place the damage. After completing this exercise, the GBT psychologist will have a short talk with the participants. intervention in which he will explain to patients where they should go to quit smoking.

Activity 8.

Theme: Healthy diet: your best option.

Contents:

1. Definition of a healthy diet.

2. Determine which foods are healthy and which are not.

Objectives:

1. To know the definition of a healthy diet.

2. Identify healthy and unhealthy foods.

3. Raise awareness of the patient's need for a healthy diet.

Time: 45 minutes

Method: Expository - Illustrative.

Media: banner.

Responsible: Principal Investigator.

Participative technique used: Didactic games.

Materials required: Table.
Procedure: In this activity, each of the patients who are participating in the intervention will be asked to bring some food, whether it is fruit, vegetables, sweets or cereals. Two tables will be set up in the classroom, each with an identification, Table 1 "Healthy foods" and Table 2 "Unhealthy foods" and they will be asked to bring their own food, either fruit, vegetables, sweets or cereals. will explain what the dynamic consists of. Each patient will choose a food item and place it on the table he/she believes it belongs to.

Activity 9.

Theme: Physical exercise. Summary:
1. Importance of regular physical exercise to improve lifestyle.
Objectives:
1. To know the importance of regular physical exercise to improve one's lifestyle.

Time: 90 minutes

Method: Expository - Illustrative. Media: banners.
Responsible: Principal Investigator.

Participatory technique used: Brainstorming.

Materials required: None.

Procedure: A discussion will be held on What is physical exercise?

How can I exercise according to my age and the pathologies I have?

How important is regular physical exercise in preventing cerebrovascular disease? After the discussion, participants will be invited to join in a healthy walk for life.

Activity 10.

Theme: Summing up what has been learned.

Contents:

• Concept of cerebrovascular diseases.

• Types, causes and symptoms of cerebrovascular diseases.
• Modifiable and non-modifiable risk factors for cerebrovascular disease.

• Importance of a healthy lifestyle.
• Farewell.

Objectives:

• To understand the concept of cerebrovascular diseases.

• Identify the types, causes and symptoms of cerebrovascular diseases.

• To know the factors of risk factors of the diseases modifiable and non-modifiable cerebrovascular diseases.

• Know the importance of leading a healthy lifestyle.

Time: 2 hours.

Method: Joint elaboration.

Media: banners, blackboard.

Responsible: Principal Investigator.

Participatory technique used: Questions and answers.

Materials required: None.

Procedure: To conclude the educational programme, a series of questions will be developed to summarise what they have learnt and to determine whether they have learnt everything about cerebrovascular diseases. They will elaborate the The participants will be divided into several groups and the most correct answer will be chosen. A toast will be made to encourage the participants in this intervention.

Annex 6. Form

- Smoking.
- High Blood Pressure (Mark with an X):
- Controlled
- Uncontrolled

Blood pressure:

- Diabetes Mellitus (Mark with an X):
- Controlled
- Uncontrolled
- Glycaemia:

TABLES

Table 1: Distribution of patients according to age group and sex. CMF Nº 11. Manuel Piti Fajardo" Teaching Polyclinic. Santo Domingo.2023.

Age group	Sex				Total	
	Female		Male			
	No.	%	No.	%	No.	%
50-54	7	20	4	11.4	11	31.4
55-60	9	25.7	15	42.8	24	68.6
Total	16	45.7	19	54.3	35	100

Table 2: Identification of risk factors for cerebrovascular disease by sex. CMF Nº 11. Manuel Piti Fajardo" Teaching Polyclinic. Santo Domingo.2023.

Risk factors for cerebrovascular disease	Sex				Total	
	Female		Male			
	No.	%	No.	%	No.	%
Ischaemic heart disease	4	11.4	6	17.1	10	28.6
Smoking	4	11.4	8	22.8	12	34.3
Arterial Hypertension	14	40.0	16	45.7	30	85.7
Diabetes Mellitus	10	28.6	8	22.8	18	51.4
History of cerebrovascular disease	1	2.8	4	11.4	5	14.3

x^2 =2.850p = 0.583

Table 3: Comparison of knowledge of types of cerebrovascular disease before and after the Education Programme. CMF Nº 11. Manuel Piti Fajardo" Teaching Polyclinic. Santo Domingo.2023.

Knowledge about types of cerebrovascular diseases	Before the Educational Programme		After the Educational Programme	
	No.	%	No.	%
Adequate	8	22.8	29	82.8
Inadequate	27	77.1	6	17.1

p = 0.001

Table 4: Comparison of knowledge of cerebrovascular disease risk factors before and after the Education Programme. CMF Nº 11. Manuel Piti Fajardo" Teaching Polyclinic. Santo Domingo.2023.

Knowledge of cerebrovascular disease risk factors	Before the Educational Programme		After the Educational Programme	
	No.	%	No.	%
Adequate	13	37.1	31	88.6
Inadequate	22	62.8	4	11.4

p = 0.002

Table 5: Comparison of High Blood Pressure before and after the Education Programme. CMF Nº 11. Manuel Piti Fajardo" Teaching Polyclinic. Santo Domingo.2023.

Arterial Hypertension	Before the Educational Programme		After the Educational Programme	
	No.	%	No.	%
Controlled	11	31.4	25	71.4
Uncontrolled	19	54.3	5	14.3

p = 0.000

Table 6: Comparison of smoking before and after the Educational Programme. CMF Nº 11. Manuel Piti Fajardo" Teaching Polyclinic. Santo Domingo.2023.

Smoking	Before the Educational Programme		After the Educational Programme	
	No.	%	No.	%
Yes	23	65.7	19	54.3
No	12	34.3	16	54.7

p = 0.009

Table 7: Comparison of Diabetes Mellitus before and after the Education Programme. CMF Nº 11. Manuel Piti Fajardo" Teaching Polyclinic. Santo Domingo.2023.

Diabetes Mellitus	Before the Educational Programme		After the Educational Programme	
	No.	%	No.	%
Controlled	10	28.6	16	45.7
Uncontrolled	8	22.8	2	5.7

p = 0.003

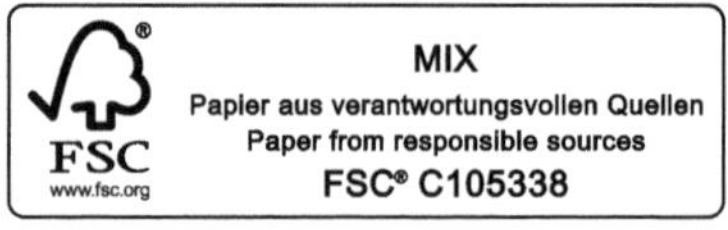

Printed by Books on Demand GmbH, Norderstedt / Germany